Is This My Child?

Sensory Integration

Simplified

Shelley Margow
MS.OTR/L

ISBN 978-1-937862-54-1

Library of Congress Control Number 2014909589

Cover design by Peter O'Connor, Bespoke Book Covers.

Published by BookCrafters,
Parker, Colorado.
http://bookcrafters.net
bookcrafters@comcast.net

This book may be ordered from
www.bookcrafters.net
and other online bookstores.

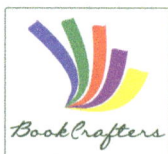

Acknowledgements

A book can be a pretty intimidating project to take on — who will actually read it? Will it make sense? and will it help someone? Regardless of these questions I have had some pretty strong supporters and without them, I would not have had the courage to go through with this.

To my wonderful husband – Andy, you have always been my biggest fan and pushed me to places that I would not have ventured to. By supporting my beliefs, you have strengthened my belief in myself and these theories which enable me to put these thoughts onto paper.

To my children who are independent, supportive young men – thank you for affording me the time to write this book and taking care of feeding yourselves.

Without the unconditional, adoring love that my parents have shown me, I would not have had the compassion, empathy and acceptance that I feel toward the parents and children that I work with. I am truly grateful for your support and guidance.

I definitely have to thank all the therapists and staff that have worked with me and for me at Children's Therapy Works for so many years. You have enabled me to learn, grow and thrive in a very challenging environment that can be highly charged and emotional. We have picked a very demanding, rewarding career – but it is well worth it when we see how many lives we change on a daily basis.

And finally, to all those parents and children that I have worked with – This book is dedicated to you. Without you, the book would never have happened. We have laughed and cried together and watched growth that restores my faith in miracles. We beat the odds, constantly. We charge against the naysayers and shape futures for children who would have been dismissed by some without a second thought – but you fought for them and so did I and I will continue to do so!

Thank you to those who believed in me and those who didn't. Life is filled with opportunities, this is one that I chose. Let's see where this path leads...

Foreword

As a pediatrician who has a large practice focused on Children with Special Health Care Needs for almost 20 years, I frequently encounter children with diagnoses related to behavior and development.

Diagnosing children who have severe problems can be easier than those with more subtle issues. You may either get told to 'wait and see,' or you may get misdiagnosed in order to fit into a particular diagnostic category and treatment regimen.

When it comes to treating developmental issues, therapy (Speech, Occupational and Physical) plays a pivotal role, sometimes for a short intensive treatment period, and sometimes for many years. Diagnosing and treating the individual correctly is crucial though, especially with Sensory Integration.

Starting with a clear and simple understanding of Sensory Integration will help understand the direction that care and therapeutic intervention needs to take. Parents and Primary Care physicians need to know how to navigate the system and move care in the right direction.

One needs an approach that takes into account the 'whole child.' This book explains just that and the approach is simple and relatable!

Kevin Berger, M.D., FAAP, FAAHPM

Kevin Berger is a general pediatrician at Phoenix Pediatrics, LTD., a private practice Medical Home that has had a strong commitment to Children with Special Health Care Needs for the past 40 years.

He is also a Pediatric Medical Director at Hospice of the Valley. His community involvement includes being a member of the Board at Ryan House as well as Hacienda Healthcare.

Table of Contents

Introduction

This is a book that has been a long time coming. I have been a Pediatric Occupational Therapist since 1994; I have watched diagnoses and therapy evolve into a myriad of labels and options. We now have statistics stating that one in 66 children have Autism, that 16% of our elementary schools are filled with children with some kind of learning disability and that stimulants are amongst the most prescribed drugs for elementary school children. Statistics are all very well and good, but what does that mean to the parent who is trying to help their child reach their highest potential, whose most accessible option is a stimulant drug? How do these statistics affect the kindergartner who can't sit still or focus on a story during a school day? The statistics provide a temporary solution. Why? Because we as parents are comfortable with the knowledge that if my child fits into a statistical group, then there must be help. If the doctors and scientists who we trust say that this is true, then it must be so.

So now I throw some questions at you: what if there is another way, and what if your child does not fit into that group and what if we, as a medical profession, have taken a word (like Autism) and made the definitions so broad, that almost any child can fit into it? And what if the label ADD or ADHD has become so well accepted that any child who cannot necessarily focus and concentrate for a certain period of time can automatically fit into this category without too much effort in finding out what the real issue is?

In this book, we will explore another way of thinking, a more fundamental principle that relates to all human beings and how a person processes, understands and uses sensory information.

I hope that in reading this book, you can walk away with practical knowledge and a variety of options that are more in tune with how the human body functions neurologically.

As humans, we evolve according to our environments, resources and genetics. It is time too that the medical and educational professions look at these factors and how they influence child development, growth and diagnosis.

When I first began treating, we saw children with specific syndromes and diagnosis: Down Syndrome, Autism (that was truly Autism), Cerebral Palsy and clear Developmental Delays and that is about it.

A child would come to therapy when they had trouble speaking and/or performing motor skills. I have watched these changes evolve into the expansion of diagnosis to cover many different areas e.g. Autism now has a full range of diagnosis such as Pervasive Developmental Disorder with modifiers added on PDD-NOS (Pervasive Developmental Disorder - Not Otherwise Specified). I could write a whole book on diagnosis but that is not the goal here. The point is to show you that we have managed to label EVERYTHING, but that doesn't necessarily mean that your child fits into that label.

We are seeing a different type of child today

— a child that can easily be diagnosed with one of the Autism diagnosis, but this child is not necessarily Autistic or on the spectrum.

This is a child who does not have severe cognitive delays, or cognitive "splinter skills." They look like their peers and are cute little munchkins who want to be a part of everything but don't know how to participate. Most likely, speech delays or differences are evident; this is the first real sign that worries parents. When we speak to the mom though, she will more often then not tell me that she knew in her gut that something was different about her child. By age four, the teachers are starting to notice differences and make comments and by second grade, the meetings with the school begin. They go something like this:

Mr. and Mrs. _____, Jonny is a very smart little boy, but he doesn't seem to be able to attend to sit down activities. He is not really applying himself. He can read, but he plays the clown when he is asked to read, or he falls off his chair a lot. He seems to avoid activities, which I know he can do. Have you spoken to your pediatrician about his attention? Maybe that would be a good idea. Translation: I believe that your child has ADHD and some medication would make him focus during class time and make him less disruptive.

The teacher is not trying to be judgmental, she truly has your child's best interests at heart, but if 10% of children between first and fifth grade are diagnosed with ADHD and 7% of those children are already on medication, then statistically it makes sense that a teacher would feel very comfortable with making that recommendation. That is just ADHD, we are not even talking about the other diagnoses out there which would affect even more children. This leads me back to the original questions of: what if we are wrong, what if there is something else going on that we have not addressed, what if there are other ways to work on the symptoms from a foundational perspective and be proactive instead of reactive? What if we as parents could make this decision and use alternatives to medication? Continue reading then and let's explore the alternatives.

This book is not intended to tell you how to raise your child or that what you are currently doing is wrong. My goal is to explore various pathways so that you can be your child's advocate and feel empowered enough to choose the path that you want to take as a parent. If I offend anyone during our journey, I apologize upfront. I am a mother of three beautiful boys and married to a wonderful man who was diagnosed with ADD at age 30. In our clinic, we have treated over 4000 families. Most of what you will read here is based on experience, research and theories that have developed from the neurological research that we have available today. All the examples and stories that you read about are real children that we have worked with; names and some circumstances are changed to protect their identities.

I hope that you walk away feeling empowered with knowledge that can help you make the right decision for you and your family.

Enjoy!

(The parental surveys revealed that a physician or psychologist had diagnosed 607 of the 6,099 children in the sample, or 10 percent, with ADHD. All of the children in the sample were first- to fifth-graders at one of the 17 public elementary schools in the county. (http://pn.psychiatryonline.org/content/37/8/46.full (http://pn.psychiatryonline.org/content/37/8/46.full). Psychiatric News April 19, 2002 vol. 37 no. 8 46-65)

An abstract of the study, prevalence of Medication Treatment for Attention-Deficit/Hyperactivity Disorder Among Elementary School Children in Johnston County, North Carolina is posted on the Web at www.ajph.org/cgi/content/abstract/92/2/231 (http://www.ajph.org/cgi/content/abstract/92/2/231).

Chapter 1

Is this my child?

James is a cute, four-and-a-half-year old who we met one summer. His parents are well-educated, successful thirty-something's living a comfortable life. James is bilingual because Mom's first language is not English. She speaks to James in her native language and Dad speaks mostly English. A few weeks after returning from our summer vacation, I received a call from Mom asking what my profession was. I explained the practice to her and my profession as an Occupational Therapist. After a brief silence, she said, "We have just been given a diagnosis of Autism." My immediate thought was no, James is not Autistic. I had spent the summer with this family. I knew that there were definitely speech-language issues and motor difficulties, but no Autism.

Through further conversations, it turned out that the psychologist had made the comment that he could look Autistic to other people and not to be surprised if he received that diagnosis but that she was not going to diagnose him with that. He flapped his hands when he was excited and spoke totally off topic when playing with his friends. The psychologist's recommendations included occupational therapy, vision therapy and speech therapy - fairly typical course of treatment for a child with these concerns.

As we continued talking, I began explaining what this all meant and the best course of action. Because we were friends, there was a trust that is not typical when talking with a new client. My friend who lived in another state packed up her stuff, got on a plane with her son and came to live in Atlanta for 25 days to attend an intensive program combining technological programs and therapy. The day before Thanksgiving, they happily hopped on a plane home, tired but rejuvenated. The best phone call that I have ever received was the following day on Thanksgiving — James' dad called me to say that James and his mom had arrived home safely and that he was so grateful to us that he did not know how to thank my team and me. Dad saw a child who could express himself clearly, he did not trip up and down the stairs, but most importantly, he had blossomed into a confident, expressive little person who made sense when he spoke and knew that he was OK, within a three-week period. He could not believe the change. Autism? No, we did not cure Autism, James was not autistic to start off with, but he very easily could have been another statistic.

Does my child do any of the following?

Let's discuss the different signs that a child like James displays. With this information, as a parent you can effectively advocate for your child.

In the introduction, I spoke about speech delays. This is the most common sign that we see fairly early on. Typical developing children have a vocabulary of four to six words by 15 months, they follow simple one step directions by 18 months and by age two should have about three simple sentences.

It concerns me when parents tell me that their children have lost speech by 18 months, because developmentally, they really shouldn't have that much speech yet, they are working on single words and the meanings of those words. Language is far more comprehensive. Receptive language develops into meaning first, so they should respond to directions and social interactions. They should be imitating their parents socially and repeating what is said. They should also be practicing certain simple words, sounds and phonemes (the unit of a sound). I have added a developmental table to show the differences in delays and typical development.

The child usually looks clumsy, they seem to have OK co-ordination and can do some activities, e.g. they may be able to ride a bike with training wheels but this is not necessarily the activity of choice. When the child goes to activities such as music or gym classes, they may not want to participate, may behave poorly or just can't seem to keep up with their peers. The child is usually resistant to participating in social activities that they inherently know is difficult for them. When they do, they appear to keep up for short periods of time then may just do their own thing or get bored and want to do something else. Many times parents will tell me that their child just didn't enjoy it so they stopped going. Well, nor would we, if we found it too challenging to do.

The next area of concern is school. I see very bright children who are set in their own ways and like to control their environments. Parents, especially mothers, accommodate their children as mother's instinct kicks in. In a classroom setting, teachers have their rules. The child has to accommodate to the classroom rules and structure and this can be very challenging when they are struggling internally. Society expects that a child will conform to their environment. Well what happens when they don't conform? We give it a name ADHD, ADD, OCD, PDD. The list goes on. This is not to say that children don't have a particular diagnosis, I want to make it clear that these are very real, effective diagnoses, I am just concerned at how quick we are to use them. I will discuss diagnoses in a later chapter.

I have briefly spoken about speech and motor delays. The third major area that we recognize is behavior difficulties. Tantrums, biting, throwing things in a stressful situation, misbehaving at the grocery store or at a birthday party. When a child behaves poorly, they are usually trying to tell us something. They are hungry, tired or just don't want to be a part of what is going on. When they are pushing the boundaries, we can use many types of discipline techniques that are mostly effective. When none of these techniques are effective, and the behavior seems unrelated to an event, or the child overreacts to a seemingly silly situation, usually there is an underlying fear or response that the brain is reacting to, and the child does not know why they have responded that way. Behaviors can manifest in anger, crying, fear, hitting, biting, kicking or not responding at all. We will talk about these behaviors in depth.

Many times I am asked, how do I know whether there is really something wrong with my child? This is my answer: When your child can't participate effectively in his/her daily functions, eating, sleeping, playing, dressing, social activities or school activities, then we have to look at why these tasks are such a struggle. If any one of these areas becomes a problem to the point that it is stressing the family or the child on a week-to-week basis, we know there is a problem.

Development is often divided into specific domains, such as gross motor; fine motor, language, cognition, and social/emotional growth. These designations are useful, but substantial overlap exists. Studies have established average ages at which specific milestones are reached, as well as ranges of neurotypical development. In a neurotypical child, progress within the different domains varies, as in the toddler who walks late but speaks in sentences early.

Here is a very basic overview of development.

Behavior

Birth
- Sleeps much of the time
- Sucks
- Clears airway
- Responds with crying to discomforts and intrusions

Four weeks
- Brings hands toward eyes and mouth
- Moves head from side to side when lying on stomach
- Follows an object moved in an arch about 15 cm above face to the midline
- Responds to a noise in some way, such as startling, crying, or quieting
- May turn toward familiar sounds and voices

Six weeks
- Regards objects in the line of vision
- Begins to smile when spoken to
- Lies flat on abdomen
- Head lags when pulled to a sitting position

Three months
- Holds head steady on sitting
- Raises head 45 degrees when lying on stomach
- Opens and shuts hands
- Pushes down when feet are placed on a flat surface
- Swings at and reaches for dangling toys
- Follows an object moved in an arc above face from one side to the other
- Watches faces intently
- Smiles at sound of caretaker's voice
- Vocalizes sounds

Five to six months
- Holds head steady when upright
- Sits with support
- Rolls over, usually from stomach to back
- Supports himself in a standing position
- Reaches for objects
- Recognizes people at a distance
- Listens intently to human voices
- Smiles spontaneously
- Squeals in delight
- Babbles to toys

Seven months
- Sits without support
- Bears some weight on legs when held upright
- Transfers objects from hand to hand
- Holds own bottle
- looks for dropped object
- Responds to own name
- Responds to being told "no"
- combines vowels and consonants to babble
- Moves body with excitement in anticipation of playing
- Plays peek-a-boo

Nine months
- Sits well
- Crawls or creeps on hands and knees
- Pulls self up to standing position
- Works to get a toy that is out of reach
- Objects if toy is taken away
- Gets into a sitting position from stomach
- Stands holding on to someone or something
- Says mama or dada appropriately in reference to parents; plays pat-a-cake
- Waves bye-bye

Twelve months
- Walks by holding furniture (cruising) or hands
- May walk one or two steps without support
- Stands for a few moments at a time
- Drinks from a cup
- Speaks several words
- Helps dress self

Eighteen months
- Walks well
- Can climb stairs holding on
- Turns several book pages at a time
- Speaks about 10 words
- Pulls toys on strings
- Partially feeds him

Two years
- Runs well
- Climbs up and down stairs alone
- Turns single book pages
- Puts on simple clothing
- Makes two or three-word sentences
- Verbalizes toilet needs

Three years
- Rides a tricycle
- Dresses well except for buttons and laces
- Counts to 10 and uses plurals
- Recognizes at least three colors
- Questions constantly
- Feeds himself well
- About one half of children can take care of toilet needs

Four years
- Alternates feet going up and down stairs
- Throws a ball overhand
- Hops on one foot
- Copies a cross
- Washes hands and face

Five years
- Skips
- Catches a bounced ball
- Copies a triangle
- Knows four colors
- Dresses and undresses without help

*   The sequence is fairly consistent, but the timing of milestones varies; times above represent median values.

As I discuss development in this book, I always take into account the whole child; therefore we look at the social, emotional, language and motor skills that are involved in development. Within the first two years of life when we see the most changes, it is important to recognize that milestones don't occur at the same time. When the brain is developing motor skills, speech skills take a back seat. When the toddler has mastered a motor skill, then the brain shifts to language development. Watching a child develop is an incredible process. It is magnificent how the brain separates skills, assimilates then integrates skills in a very logical, well-rounded manner. This is why development is so varied. When you understand how all the pieces are created then organized and fitted together like a puzzle, it is fairly easy to recognize difficulties.

During the interview process with parents, Mom, more often then not, will tell me that she had a gut feeling that something didn't feel right but she could not pin-point what it was. There was nothing really visible or tangible that she could vocalize. Mostly, Mom would get these kinds of responses: "Oh stop you're being silly; your child is just fine." Or "Don't worry, your child will grow out of it." This is one of the worst sayings that I hear only too often. Children do not grow out of anything, their bodies adapt! Depending on how they adapt determines how they eventually learn. If the adaptive mechanism is efficient and effective, then the child works through their skills without excessive effort. When the adaptive mechanism is not efficient or effective, we see dysfunction, sometimes much later on.

I called this chapter: *Is this my child?* because I hear this on a daily basis. "You have described my child or how do you know, you haven't seen my child yet?" There are many features that may describe your child.

The following check list may help determine whether to continue reading or not.

Child's Name:

_____

Today's date:

_____

Form completed by:

_____

Relationship to child:

_____

SENSORY PROCESSING SCREENING CHECKLIST

This checklist was designed to be a quick screening tool for sensory processing deficits. Please indicate if your child always responds or greater than 50% of the time responds. If several items are checked throughout many categories or most items are checked in one category, sensory processing deficits may be present.

Tactile Processing (sense of touch)
☐ bothered by clothing tags/textures
☐ refuses to wear shoes/socks
☐ avoids messy play (glue,paint)
☐ refuses to play in sand at beach
☐ hates haircuts, nail trim, tooth brush
☐ reacts neg. to touch/pulls away
☐ unaware of pain or temp.
☐ prefers to touch vs be touched
☐ withdraws from splashing water
☐ revs up after bath
☐ rubs/scratches where touched
☐ mouths clothing/objects
☐ overly fidgets/tugs at clothing
☐ does not like hands dirty

Auditory Processing (hearing)
☐ covers ears at loud noises
☐ upset with vacuum, hairdryer,toilet
☐ difficulty following directions
☐ appears to ignore name called
☐ unaware speaks too loudly
☐ distracted by background noises
☐ notices noises usually tuned out
☐ difficulty eating in noisy places
☐ slow to respond to verbal cues
☐ escapes from noisy places

Visual Processing (vision)
☐ poor eye contact
☐ likes to stare at shiny/spinning things
☐ prefers dark/ avoids bright sunlight
☐ turns whole body to look at you
☐ squints/covers eyes in sunlight
☐ covers/closes one eye when writing
☐ prefers fast paced tv shows
☐ misinterprets facial expressions
☐ illegible writing
☐ difficulty copying from the board

Proprioception (position sense)
☐ overly rough in play
☐ seems to enjoy crashing
☐ jumps from unsafe heights/jumps a lot
☐ holds pencil too hard
☐ appears clumsy/ poor coordination
☐ moves stiffly
☐ slouches at desk or table
☐ fatigues quickly
☐ prefers sedentary play
☐bumps into others/pushes others
☐ uses too much force to throw or kick

Vestibular (movement sense)
☐ on the go/trouble sitting still at table
☐ twirls self during the day; fidgets

- [ ] does not appear to get dizzy
- [ ] afraid of heights
- [ ] seeks out swinging or climbing more than typical
- [ ] poor safety awareness/ use of caution
- [ ] avoids movement on playground
- [ ] fearful with head tipped back during bath or diaper change
- [ ] afraid of elevators or escalators
- [ ] leans on others for support when sitting or standing
- [ ] moves slowly on uneven surfaces
- [ ] loses balance easily
- [ ] becomes overly excited w/movement

Oral Processing (taste)
- [ ] picky eater (refuses food due to temp or texture)
- [ ] gags at/on foods or utensils
- [ ] hates tooth brushing
- [ ] bites/chews on nonfood items
- [ ] avoids foods that require lots of chew
- [ ] craves certain foods/textures

Olfactory (sense of smell)
- [ ] smells everything
- [ ] bothered by smells others do not notice
- [ ] refuses food based on smell

Behavior

- ☐ difficulty with transitions/ changes in routine
- ☐ poor frustration tolerance
- ☐ impulsive; poor self control
- ☐ overly emotional or sensitive
- ☐ frequent tantrums/meltdowns
- ☐ unable to calm self after tantrum
- ☐ difficulty sleeping thru the night
- ☐ difficulty getting started with tasks

Social Skills

- ☐ difficulty making or maintaining friendships
- ☐ unable to interpret social cues
- ☐ does not understand age appropriate jokes
- ☐ unable to sympathize with others
- ☐ easily upset by criticism
- ☐ tries to control others/bossy
- ☐ does not share easily/take turns
- ☐ does not respect personal space of others

ADL/Play skills

- ☐ difficulty completing grooming or dressing in reasonable time/skill
- ☐ difficulty using eating utensils

- ☐ unable to manage clothing fasteners
- ☐ difficulty following or copying gestures
- ☐ does not prefer or play with age appropriate toys

Chapter 2

Understanding how the body works

The truth about developmental milestones:

Watching an infant develop over the first year of life is nothing but miraculous. This helpless little being blossoms into a laughing little cherub that explores its environment with constant amazement and wonder. Their learning and growth is literally constant with sounds, smells, touch and movement evolving into useful functional skills that we call developmental milestones. A little one's curiosity is an innate neurological function that allows the brain to experience new and previously learned experiences. It then co-ordinates, sifts out and creates new pathways that further foster development.

Developmental milestones don't just happen automatically. They are a combination of the senses and systems that efficiently co-ordinate and redirect information until the outcome seems right.

Lets look at some examples: When a child first learns to breast feed, they are programmed to instinctually find the nipple and suck. But this is one of the most difficult processes in the western world today. We all know the benefits of breastfeeding but it is a skill that none of us as mothers have performed before. We feel like it should be natural and we should know how to just do it and yet most of us give up after two weeks of struggling to performing this seemingly simple task. Breastfeeding is anything but simple or convenient. In the first month it can be excruciatingly painful, it changes our body image and it feels as if we have become a milk factory rather then a loving earth mother who cuddles her new born thereby providing safety and nourishment. In truth, it is just as hard for this helpless little thing to know what to do as much as it is for us.

An infant has to learn how to suck on a nipple whilst we are learning to reorganize our internal belief system of how we think this process should work. Not how it actually does work.

A baby sucks in utero, we sometimes are privileged enough to see this via a scan when they suck their little thumbs. In fact, they suck continuously whilst in this fluid environment. When they leave the comfort of the womb, the newborn has to adapt to having a different shaped object in their mouth and actually draw nutrition from it an instinctual knowledge. What is learned and not reliant on instinct is how to suck. Initially the infant has a negative pressure suck that allows the tongue to push the nipple to the roof of the mouth, forcing the milk to squirt to the back of the throat then slide down the throat. As the process gets easier the process shifts and the infant gains more control over how much milk is released into the mouth and a swallow progresses to a more mature suck, swallow and breathe synchrony.

This very integrated, complex process is the basic foundation for setting up eating patterns for the rest of the baby's life. An infant that struggles with the suck-swallow-breathe synchrony is the picky-eater that we see later on in life. Reflux can be a symptom of a very poor suck-swallow-breathe synchrony. This is a huge issue that we see today and one of the issues that are often seen in the developmental history questionnaire that parents complete when they come for evaluations when a child is much older — four and up. The common fix — Prevacid — a drug tested on adults, not infants.

My point with this example is that from the very beginning whether it is breast or bottle feeding, it is absolutely crucial that an infant develop an appropriate suck-swallow-breathe. This also forms the basis for developing appropriate breathing, sleeping and eating mechanisms. An infant that eats well and comfortably, generally has decent sleeping patterns and is more alert during the day. They adapt to transitions easier, which make for happier days because they tend to go with the flow. That is not to say that this happens all the time — children are still children and just as we think we have figured them out, something changes. This information provides a common sense guide to good health and wellness for the child and family unit.

I have spent some time describing this initial process because it plays a significant role in sensory motor development. Sensory motor development and sensory integration play a very important role in overall motor coordination, speech development and creating the foundations for further neurological development. By laying down these strong foundations, the different areas of the brain begin to work together succinctly and efficiently. The neurological pathways form cohesive mechanisms to support them rather then adapting to a less efficient process, which leads to maladaptive development.

Chapter 3

Sensory Integration: the simple version

As the infants develop, they begin to explore their environments through sensory experiences. They have a fascination with new, exciting experiences using touch to explore texture, form, shapes; proprioception and vestibular processing to explore body awareness and movement in relation to body position in space; auditory processing skills to understand sound and it's relationship to movement and spatial relationships, understanding verbal language; vision to relay all the information surrounding them. The visual system also acts as a continual reminder of whether the body is experiencing what it is seeing. Do the other senses match what the eyes are seeing and interpreting. Does the information match between all senses or are there mismatches somewhere along the line. The movement system is a complex combination of how we integrate vision, joint position and movement.

This exploration is critical in creating the future pathways for learning and development.

Learning does not occur without input of all kinds. The ability to learn is dependent on how the brain interprets information. This is clearly seen in thousands of studies relating to people who have had traumatic brain injuries and strokes. Before the insult to the brain, they could do everything they needed to without having to think about it. After the injury they have to relearn everything and may have to learn different ways of doing things with certain types of equipment and adaptive mechanisms.

Child development is assumed and we assume that our children just know how to do things. The brain is a wonderful computer — it is highly intuitive and will automatically send information to the rest of the body to perform a function. The truth is that the brain relies on internal and external information. The internal information is how the nerves are sending the messages to the brain. The outside information is how the brain is perceiving and relaying environmental stimulation to the relevant areas so that it can move to an internal process. The combination of both internal and external stimuli creates the necessary actions that facilitate child development. We are familiar with all the charts, internet resources and checklists that tell us what the developmental milestones are. We also watch all the developmental programs on TV channels that promise to teach your child to read, write etc. I am always amazed that we don't see programs that teach us to play with our children and foster their connections between the internal and external world. By doing this we inherently watch the development of language skills.

So what is Sensory Integration ....? Really?

Sensory Integration is a term that was described by Dr. Jean Ayres in the late 1960s in her book called *Sensory Integration and the Child*. She describes the theory in three parts: 1. the theory of sensory integration, 2. the evaluation and 3. the treatment.

The term itself is really very clever because that's what the brain does — it takes all this information from the five senses, integrates and interprets the information and then creates a response. The response is typically where we see the breakdown, but remember, the response contains a complex combination of inputs, planning, energy and throughput.

We have used the following pyramid to visually describe how this all works.

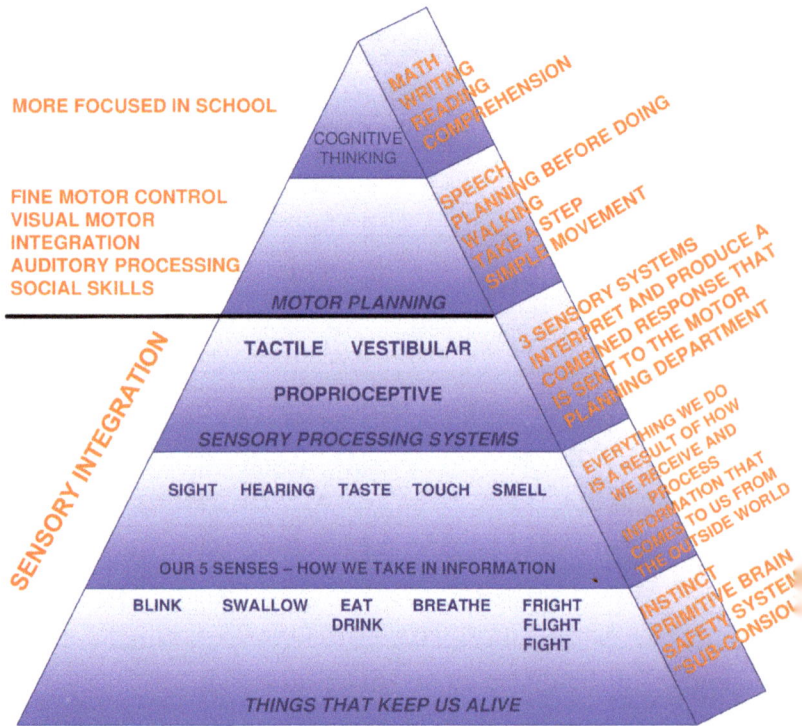

MORE FOCUSED IN SCHOOL

FINE MOTOR CONTROL
VISUAL MOTOR
INTEGRATION
AUDITORY PROCESSING
SOCIAL SKILLS

MATH
WRITING
READING
COMPREHENSION

COGNITIVE
THINKING

SPEECH
PLANNING BEFORE DOING
WALKING
TAKE A STEP
SIMPLE MOVEMENT

MOTOR PLANNING

TACTILE   VESTIBULAR

PROPRIOCEPTIVE

SENSORY PROCESSING SYSTEMS

3 SENSORY SYSTEMS
INTERPRET AND PRODUCE A
COMBINED RESPONSE THAT
IS SENT TO THE MOTOR
PLANNING DEPARTMENT

SENSORY INTEGRATION

SIGHT   HEARING   TASTE   TOUCH   SMELL

OUR 5 SENSES – HOW WE TAKE IN INFORMATION

EVERYTHING WE DO
IS A RESULT OF HOW
WE RECEIVE AND
PROCESS
INFORMATION THAT
COMES TO US FROM
THE OUTSIDE WORLD

| BLINK | SWALLOW | EAT DRINK | BREATHE | FRIGHT FLIGHT FIGHT |

INSTINCT
PRIMITIVE BRAIN
SAFETY SYSTEM
SUB-CONSCIOUS

THINGS THAT KEEP US ALIVE

The first three levels of this pyramid involve neurological functions that are somewhat programmed in the brain at a very deep level. The first level involves limbic processes that keep us alive through instinct. This "lizard" brain senses danger and its job is to keep us out of harm. These processes tend to be automatic. The blink, swallow and breathing functions are all reflexive and necessary to ensure that the body functions normally. Eating and drinking are motor skills that are governed by hunger and thirst, deeply automated processes that preserve life. *Flight-fright-fight* is commonly known as functions of the lizard brain or animalistic part of our brains that protect us from danger.

The second level of the pyramid consists of the five senses. This involves receiving sensory information through specific nerves that are attached to organs: sight=eyes; hearing=ears; taste=tongue; touch=skin; smell=nose. We all learned about the functions of these organs in school at some point in time. However we did not learn about the three systems that co-ordinate all this information.

This is the third level: vestibular, tactile and proprioceptive systems. These systems are essential in being able to co-ordinate the senses into a sensible manner. In order to function efficiently, each system requires at least two senses, e.g. the vestibular system needs to receive information from the ears and the eyes to understand movement. The tactile system typically uses many more senses e.g. smell, taste, touch, pressure. There are so many complex receptors in the eyes and ears that scientists still don't know how it works, we just know that it all has to work together to perform the necessary function.

The tactile system uses information from the skin, mouth and all the little receptors in the skin (which is the largest organ our body has). Its main job is to receive physical information from the environment and interpret the information by filtering out what to attend to, how to respond to the input and where to send it next. The signals create a complex web of information that initially determines whether the body is safe. Once safety is assessed, it then moves to a higher level in the brain to figure out what kind of response is required. e.g. when you are fearful, the hair on the back of your neck may stand up, you become alert, blood flow shifts to move to your muscles in case you have to run and all other non essential functions such as digestion slows down. Another example is when you feel an insect, on your skin, if you have a fear of spiders, your response may immediately shift to panic — your body responds with rapid, flailing movements, you may scream and jump and definitely try to get rid of this massive attack on your persona!

What we see in our children is more long term and maybe less dramatic, but these "out of context" behaviors may be something that we see in a child with an over sensitive tactile system.

The vestibular system controls and co-ordinates head and eye movements in relation to body information and movement through space. The vestibular system co ordinates and integrates how the eyes, ears and cerebellum (lower part of the brain) work together. In order to understand this, lets do a little anatomy lesson.

The ear has two functions: it receives information as sound waves and transmits the sound to the brain as a nerve impulse. The second function is for the sense of balance. We know that an ear infection makes you feel dizzy, that's because the fluid in the ear gets thick and yucky, making it difficult for the fluid to move through the semi-circular canals easily.

The semi-circular canals are key components in providing the brain with the information needed to keep your head in various positions and maintaining balance. Why is this so important you ask? Well the vestibular system controls and manages how we learn to move, making it a key component in child development. This system provides the building blocks for motor development. If the vestibular system is not functioning optimally, we see slower motor and speech development, which in turn affects all levels of higher cognitive learning.

The proprioceptive system controls joint position in space. This system guides all movements that occur at the joints and plays a role in developing how we interpret prepositions in language. If you don't know that your hand is "up" internally, then how do you understand what the word "up" means. This translates into many more play related circumstances such as going "up" and "down" a ladder at the park. When mommy says "come down" from the play equipment, if the brain is busy focusing on something else, it may completely miss the word resulting in an "unwanted" behavior. When mommy panics because her child is "not listening," he reads her body language and expressions (visual system taking over) and then assumes that he did something very wrong. Can you see how this "mis-communication" creates a potentially challenging situation in a public place?

We have to look at these three systems and understand how they affect all levels of development. By doing so, it helps us identify the "whys" of some of the issues that we see in both our diagnosed and undiagnosed children today.

It is important to understand that these three systems rely completely on each other to provide the brain with the most usable information. If one of these systems is out of balance, the other two are immediately affected! So when a child has an ear infection, or 20, the vestibular system is compromised which in turn affects the other two systems. This causes inefficient processing resulting in maladaptive responses to the environment.

All skills above this level are learnt. Once the brain sends the information to the different areas of the brain, skills develop; first on a basic level and then become more complex. We all have to learn to walk, talk and interact with the environment and people. We learn these skills usually in a step-by-step manner called motor planning. Most all skills require a component of movement, language, emotion and memory. When we put these all together, the brain becomes efficient at learning new skills.

Chapter 4

Let's put this all together

In chapter three I explained very briefly how the brain takes in information and creates a response, what I'll discuss with you in this chapter is how it all relates to the human experience.

What makes us different to every other living thing is how we experience our environments and use that to create learning, both positive and negative. There is plenty of information out there about human intelligence and what separates us from our animal counterparts. Sometimes I wonder whether our animal friends are smarter then us. They respond to dangerous situations, they rely on senses and instinct to make decisions and they don't let emotions make up their minds for them. Who is better off? As adults I'm sure many of you have looked at your sleeping dog or cat and thought "man, what a life, no stress, all you do is sleep, run after squirrels, eat, pee and poop" ... I know that I have!

But that is what makes us so incredibly unique and amazing. We do think for ourselves, we are able to interpret and understand what is happening around us and we really do rely on memory and emotion to create our own experiences.

When I first started treating, I had a hard time explaining this concept to parents. People would tell me that I was "too high level" and they could not understand the convoluted way in which I was trying to explain how the brain worked and what that meant for their child. It was all too confusing. I had to figure out a way to make this process simple and relatable.

For weeks, I threw ideas onto large pieces of paper and finally figured out a kind of a formula. SO here goes, this is the crux of how children learn from a sensory integration perspective.

The brain relies on memory to relate to an experience. If this is a new experience, then it has to form a new neurological pathway and this takes a good amount of energy.

If we think of how we process information, we could use this formula to break down the components of healthy sensory integration.

Let's start backwards. We understand ourselves in terms of communication, beliefs and interactions.

Communication incorporates the following:

The awareness of communication
The power of communication
Non-verbal communication
Verbal communication

The awareness of communication is the very first step in understanding that there is an interaction with the outside world. This occurs in utero when the baby responds to voices and noises. The brain is responding to sound. Once the brain is aware of communication, it begins to decide how to use communication skills through verbal and non-verbal cues and skills which leads to understanding how powerful communication is.

When a child has not figured out that communication gives them power, they struggle finding their voice and usually find other ways of making their needs and wants known. This can manifest as meltdowns, behavior outburst or just ignoring the different types of stimuli coming into the body.

Our belief systems develop around our basic needs and instincts, and internal and external beliefs.

Basic needs and instincts are controlled in the limbic system (or lizard brain). This is the area of the brain that keeps us out of harm's way. It is the *flight-fright-fight* part of the brain which controls and balances many different chemicals that help keep us feeling safe and secure. Without this sense of security, the brain can remain on alert for unspecified amounts of time, which becomes a very unhealthy, unbalanced way to live. When there is chemical imbalance, there is

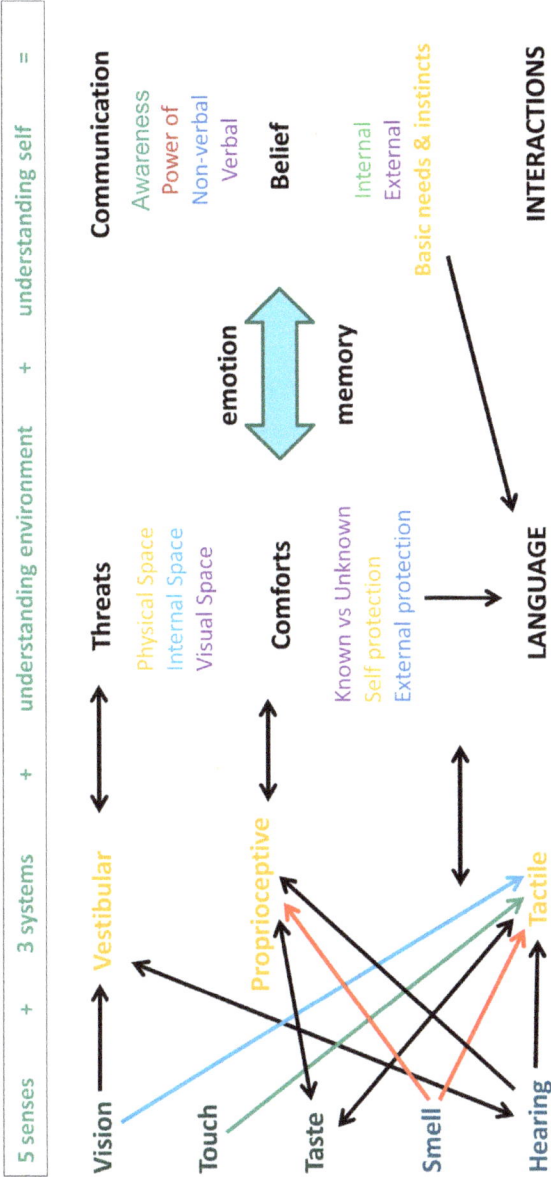

5 senses + 3 systems + understanding environment + understanding self =

Communication
Awareness
Power of
Non-verbal
Verbal

Belief
Internal
External
Basic needs & instincts

INTERACTIONS

emotion

memory

Threats
Physical Space
Internal Space
Visual Space

Comforts
Known vs Unknown
Self protection
External protection

LANGUAGE

Vision

Touch

Taste

Smell

Hearing

Vestibular

Proprioceptive

Tactile

A WHOLE CHILD

an energetic shift in where impulses in the brain go. This *flight-fright-fight* response is supposed to be temporary, but when it becomes part of the daily function of the brain, the ability to perform higher level processes becomes hindered. There is only so much energy that can be used and accessed at a time.

Our external belief system has a very powerful affect on how we perceive who we are. Our environment and how people treat us affect these beliefs. If a child is taught early on in life that they are "bad," then they believe this to be true and act accordingly — which may be completely maladaptive. This external belief system then internalizes to become truth in the brain. The brain itself cannot distinguish between what is real and what is perceived. I'm sure you have heard the saying: "Your perception becomes your belief which becomes your reality."

The subconscious mind of a child is completely under-developed and brand new! It is wide open to the possibilities and if those possibilities are negative, then that is what develops in the subconscious brain.

These belief systems influence and drive communication skills, which are influenced by interactions with others, the environment and oneself to become a complex, woven pattern of events, behaviors and learning.

Once these patterns develop, they rely on memory and emotion to lay down neurological pathways in the brain. These pathways start as simple patterns that are practiced and modified depending on the responses that are received through understanding self and understanding the environment.

We understand our environment in terms of threats, comforts and language (language is different from communication).

We understand and perceive threats in terms of physical space, internal space and visual space. I have specifically divided these into these three areas because of where the brain sends all this information.

An example of physical space is our own personal space around us. We learn through our cultural influences what is acceptable personal space and what isn't. We are taught that we do not enter someone else's physical space, which consists of an arms length around us (western culture).

Our internal space is our intuitive sense of our own body — what feels threatening to us, feelings of hunger, tiredness, needing to use the bathroom. When this internal space is threatened, the brain automatically moves into a sense of *flight-fright-fight* again. We find internal ways of protecting ourselves. If someone is feeling depressed, you may find it difficult to get out of bed and want to stay snuggled up under the covers to protect yourself.

A child who feels this internal threat may not want to be held by anyone but his or her mother. This is then seeking external comfort.

Visual threats are exactly that — what I see appears dangerous and I need to remove myself from the situation. The best example that I can offer is this: one of the most common goals that I see on a therapy report is — "child will make eye contact!" To me that is one of the most insulting goals to see on a report. Visual space is the one thing that all children have control over. When a child is struggling to make eye contact, there is a much deeper reason then, "he doesn't want to look at me." It's usually related to perceiving the visual space as a threat and the brain switches into this *flight-fright-fight* response (which I have only mentioned about 50 times in the last few pages). The automatic response from the visual system neurologically is to switch to using the peripheral visual fields. This allows the body the freedom to flee and see what options it has to move - which space it can move to. When the brain remains in this state, the cortical visual fields take a back seat. Cortical visual fields are what we use to learn to read, write and participate in activities that are within our internal sense of space.

These two visual fields rely on each other to switch from learning mode to "what is going on around me" mode. The child who continually day dreams is living in peripheral visual mode — ADD? Hhhmmm.

Understanding our environments in terms of comforts allows the body to differentiate between known and unknown comforts, self protection and external protection.

Known vs unknown comforts are always an interesting concept to me. Infants learn to soothe themselves using various techniques such as sucking a pacifier, or their thumb, being held and rocked or as they get older, seeking tangible objects such as their blanket or favorite fluffy toy.

If a child is not able to self soothe, they may rely more on self protection and external protection. Self protection may include tantrums or crying, whereas external protection may be hanging on fiercely to mommy's leg and not letting go for ANYTHING.

These threats and comforts create the stage for language development. Now note, I did not say communication, I want to reiterate that communication does not require language, but language is a clear form of communication.

When we understand our environments and self, using emotion and memory loops, the brain continues to weave solid foundations of development. As the brain develops and grows, further patterns become automatic and allow for higher level learning.

When there is a traffic jam in any of these patterns and the flow of energy is interrupted for whatever reason, then the patterns of development become maladaptive and we see the symptoms of this in behaviors, motor and speech development, and learning.

By tracing back to where the underlying problems or interruptions are, there is usually a very clear glitch in one or more of the sensory systems that we spoke about in chapter three. As I discussed, all three systems work together to create balance in the body and brain. The job of these three systems is to assist the brain in understanding the self and the environment.

The vestibular system influences the brains perception on understanding space. The vestibular system controls and integrates visual, auditory and movement — providing the necessary stimuli to understand physical, internal and visual space (understanding the environment in terms of threats).

The proprioceptive system controls comforts. Most people feel safe when receiving a hug. This is the proprioceptive and tactile system kicking in — deep pressure creates a sense of safety. The tactile system warns us against noxious stimuli.

The proprioceptive system provides understanding language, prepositions and understanding of oneself.

So you can see that these three systems are the foundational components for the development of understanding the environment and oneself.

By using these constant patterns, our memories and emotions develop as well.

Every memory is linked to an emotion and a sense. Think about a situation that brought you comfort as a child — it may be standing in the kitchen watching your grandma make muffins. Do you remember the warmth of the kitchen, the smell of baking, and your feeling of contentment?

Now think back to a challenging experience. Maybe a teacher who you didn't like, the musty odor of the classroom and how you felt during that time. Even though you're an adult now, those memories are still deeply embedded in your brain.

Let's reverse the game — when you walk into a room and smell a familiar perfume, what memory does that smell trigger?

You get my point, senses create memories,

which relate to emotions. Emotions integrate sensations with memories.

This is very powerful!

As the brain becomes more proficient at processing this information, these patterns get stored away, getting deeper and deeper as the brain needs them less and less. The processes become automatic and integrated.

When there is inefficient processing, instead of integrating and storing this information, the nerve impulses become inefficient and get used in various ways that then begin to form maladaptive responses which requires even more energy, leaving less available power for higher levels of learning. So what does this all look like in our children?

Chapter 5

How does Sensory Integration affect our children?

As discussed in earlier chapters, Sensory Integration is a term that we use to describe how the brain interprets, processes and produces an output in relation to self and the environment.

Efficient sensory integration provides an integrated, adaptive response to learning and integrating new skills as well as being able to use previously learned skills effectively for learning.

Sensory integration affects motor skills, language, social skills and higher academic learning.

All human beings process information — sensory integration occurs every second of the day in every human brain. It is not some high-in-the-sky phenomena that are difficult to understand.

Yes this is a neurological process that lays down patterns of information using complex, neuroplasticity to develop a well rounded, healthy brain that is able to access the necessary tools required for learning.

Environmental stresses, nutrition, hydration and movement influence sensory integration.

It is not a disease or genetic disorder. Some consider it a mental health issue. I personally disagree with that because there is so much research and information available to us on brain function and how the nervous system translates information through the various brain waves.

In this chapter, I want to talk about how disruptions in sensory processing affect our kids and the relationship this has to diagnoses.

My intention is to simplify and outline the primary factors that affect children with these diagnoses, then add the sensory integration component to explain what the potential foundational concerns are.

Autism

The child with an Autism/PDD/ Asperger's diagnosis primarily has difficulty connecting socially with people. They may have difficulties with interpreting social cues, facial expressions, voice intonations and body language overall.

Most of these kids also have some pretty stand-out sensory processing difficulties such as slow motor co-ordination development, being picky eaters, disliking the feel of clothing or shoes, showers or having their hair washed. Self stimulating behaviors or obsessing over a particular object such as lining toys up, trains or vehicles of some kind.

It is not unusual for us, as clinicians, to see secondary diagnoses such as ADD/ADHD, obsessive compulsive disorders, gastric disorders and reflux and the list goes on.

ADD/ADHD

Is a diagnosis given to a child when their daily function is hindered by lack of focus and attention. Attention Deficit Disorder (ADD) does not have the hyperactive component that the ADHD has; meaning that the child with ADD usually day dreams in class, forgets what they are working on and generally has a low level of engagement in the classroom — but can play video games for hours on end.

The child with ADHD, generally has a hard time staying still and moves constantly in the environment disrupting classmates and generally not getting the necessary work done.

Kids with ADD/ADHD can be extremely smart with high IQ scores and can have some pretty interesting behaviors.

Non-verbal Learning Disability

This is a very interesting diagnosis and looks very similar to Autism in the early years. We don't see this diagnosis much because so many of our kids get the autism diagnosis instead. Kids with NVLD learn fast and with the right interventions no longer appear autistic after about age five to six. I often wonder to myself whether these are the kids whose parents or professionals view them as "cured" from autism.

I need to add here, that I don't believe autism is a disease — therefore it does not need to be cured. No don't worry, you don't have to get so upset — but the research is definitely showing that there are genetic markers in the DNA of children with autism. Just like Down Syndrome is not a disease, nor is Autism — these are beautiful, perfect children who we honor and admire for their strength and what they teach us as human beings! So there, I have said my piece, I will now get back to the matter at hand.

SPD - Sensory Processing Disorder

Is a real diagnosis! We (clinicians) usually use it as a secondary diagnosis because it has not been officially accepted in the medical model. I can tell you however that it is very real.

SPD is used when the child has been seen by an Occupational Therapist who has done the Sensory Integration and Praxis Test, and or the Sensory Profile (or any of the other standardized tests that measure these skills); and determined that there is a definite breakdown in how these three systems are processing and integrating information.

Dyspraxia

Dyspraxia is a functional diagnosis that occurs when an obviously bright child is struggling to learn new skills in either the motor or speech areas or both. The child with dyspraxia can also look like a child with autism. The big difference is that they connect with people and the environment. The child wants positive feedback from parents and teachers and they try really hard to make their needs and wants known.

So here comes the challenge! Many of the children that come to us for therapy can have one or all of these diagnoses. What I find interesting however, is that depending on who diagnosed the child, will depend on the type of treatment they receive. Well that seems like quite an obvious statement, but the obvious statement to me would be that any child and parent going through an evaluation process should have access to the information that will create the most comprehensive treatment protocol for that family. But that is not happening. So hopefully, this little book will offer some options that can empower parents and children alike.

So we ask the question again about how sensory integration affects our children.

It's pretty simple in my mind — we can look at the diagnosis as a whole or we can look at the symptomology, which tends to overlap between all these diagnoses.

The first thing to consider is this *flight-fight-fright* response. I have spoken a lot about this because it is the first thing that we have to determine when looking at our children. Do they feel safe? A child with Autism struggles with communication (not just language but all the levels of communication that were discussed in previous chapters). Communication gives us power and control — well if you can't control and understand your environment, then you live in constant survival mode, not knowing what to expect next.

A child with ADD or ADHD is so used to being reprimanded and/or corrected, that they have learnt to either suppress emotion or "behave badly." This occurs because their interpretation of the world is so completely different, that they just react and respond impulsively and emotionally. Their belief systems become skewed, and their trust in the world dwindles — back to the *flight-fright-fight* response.

I think you are getting the picture here.

So really any one of these diagnoses is just providing a tangible name to group a cluster of symptoms together. The problem with this is the child then becomes a lab experiment for medications — yes, I know that is very harsh, but unfortunately true.

Don't get me wrong here, medication has its place and can be highly effective, but it should be the last resort, not the first.

By understanding how the brain processes information and using those tools as a treatment technique, we are able to address the underlying issues that are creating the end result.

Let's look at some examples:

Victor was four years old when I first saw him in my office. He had come to see me because he had been asked to leave a Montessori preschool due to behavior issues. His parents were at their wits' end and didn't know where to turn. My first encounter with Victor was coaxing him out from under the desk in the evaluation room...except that he wouldn't budge, so we just worked like that until he felt safe enough to not need this external safety net (the table). When I tested Victor, his testing scores indicated a VERY bright child with major visual perceptual difficulties, an over-sensitive vestibular and tactile system and an under-responsive proprioceptive system.

We started intensive therapy fairly quickly using a variety of neurological programs in combination with occupational, physical and speech therapies. Within about six months, Victor had learned that communication was power and as he began to understand his own body, he became more comfortable with the environment and himself, lessening the

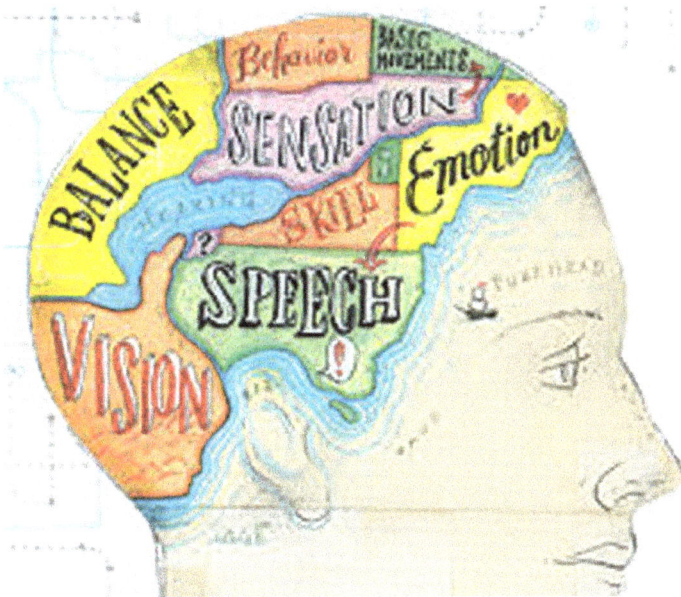

behaviors and break downs significantly. As we peeled the layers of the onion away, the deeper issues began to arise. We quickly figured out that Victor had severe auditory defensiveness, so we gave him head phones (that he chose) that he could use to block out the unbearable sounds whenever he needed to. Victor had always been extremely sedentary, so we had to get him moving to encourage the necessary vestibular processing that would "feed" the brain to understand movement. As these skills developed, Victor's confidence and belief in himself blossomed. We started to see a little boy who was OK with his world —yes, there were some pretty harrowing days, but with time, attention to his needs and the necessary input, his brain moved out of *flight-fright-fight* and into learning mode.

But Victor was still struggling to learn reading skills. We had worked in rhythm, timing and sequencing, we had continued with sensory integration treatment and yet he was still struggling with visual perceptual activities. So we sent Victor for a developmental vision assessment and what we found explained so much! Victor had a severe case of convergence insufficiency! In other words, he saw double ... all the time, so asking his cortical visual skills to focus on a book or the board was just impossible. Treatment shifted to working on these issues and within another six months or so, Victor started reading. During this time, we had started a school for children who just didn't fit anywhere else. We weren't concerned about their diagnosis or there behaviors. The goal of the school was to use this sensory integration philosophy, together with neurological programming, speech and social skills and play based activities to facilitate appropriate learning.

Victor attended the Academy for two years and successfully mainstreamed into public school. We were all so proud! Victor continues to receive Equine Assisted Psychotherapy as an outlet for his emotional and social development and is about to do another intensive summer program in the clinic.

I am very grateful to Victor and his parents for giving me the opportunity to learn from his struggles as well as giving hope to other families out there who may be experiencing similar struggles.

Chapter 6

So, what do we do about it?

Sensory Integration treatment is a highly specialized field. When I started learning about this early on in my career, we had to whisper the word — it was voodoo, nonsense, made no sense to the average doctor, etc. etc. The fact is today it is a well accepted, researched theory and form of treatment, it is just not marketed.

We have a vast knowledge of autism, ADD/ADHD, OCD, Bipolar Disorders and Depression because the pharmaceutical companies have such a financial hold on the market. Medication is a quick fix, its easy to access, easy to administer and promises immediate results. But what happens when it doesn't work for your child? What are the options then?

Therapy is highly specialized and expensive. It is not a quick fix and it requires emotional, financial and time investments from the entire family. But the big difference between this type of intervention and medication, is that sensory integration and neurological therapies work and change the brain's processing ability for the long term. It is not a temporary fix — it is powerful enough to change the chemistry of the brain through neuroplasticity.

Neuroplasticity simply put is the brain's ability to recreate new synapses and neural pathways that allow for growth and development. In children, the brain is incredibly pliable and open to learning, which makes working with these kiddies such a joy.

Children learn through play. Many times when I do new evaluations now, we are not seeing children play and use their imaginations like they used to. This could be another whole book — yes TV, video games and technology definitely play a role in children not moving as much as they used to, however this is only one area affecting our kids today.

Play has become static — hmm, that's a contradiction. Look at our playgrounds today — nothing moves except the swings, and even those are restricted to a certain height. In the name of safety, we have removed the most important pieces of equipment from our play grounds — really tall, straight slides, with high ladders and deep, sudden drops. Merry-go-rounds and seesaws. Think about what these types of experiences taught us — "it was frightening climbing up that tall ladder to get to the top of the slide, but once I went sliding down, it was exhilarating!" Engaging and experimenting with this play equipment taught us safety skills, (you better know where to put your foot on the ladder because it's a long way down!). The merry-go-round encouraged us to run really fast other wise we weren't going to make it on to the platform — this taught the brain spatial relationships, body awareness in space, visual space management, strength in the upper body, bilateral Co-ordination in the lower limbs, timing and sequence and of course feeling dizzy after the spinning stopped. Who would have thought that such a simple exercise was so powerful.

That's what sensory integration treatment is all about. A well trained therapist assesses and recognizes the underlying processes that are causing and creating the presenting difficulties in a child; then uses play (a child's occupation) to retrain the neural networks. By providing play experiences that are engaging, movement based, safe and experiential; the child is able to trust their own skills, opening up the possibility for exploration and learning how to trust their own bodies leading to meaningful relationships with their internal sense of self, their environment and others.

In children with the autism diagnoses, we see social, language and motor difficulties.

In children with ADD/ADHD, attention, concentration and behavior struggles.

All these children regardless of diagnosis show sensory processing difficulties, whether it's behavioral, language based or motor based, or possibly all three, they will ALL benefit from sensory integration treatments.

Chapter 7

Intensive Step up Approach to Intervention

Sensory Integration treatment can be a confusing mish mush of swings and equipment. Parents have told me many times that their child is doing SI treatment one time a week. When I ask them specifically what their child does in treatment, they tell me things like "they sit on a swing for about 10 minutes of the session then work on coloring." This is not SI treatment, it may be adequate occupational therapy, but it is definitely not SI.

In order for Sensory Integration treatment to be effective, it has to be done consistently and intensely for a period of time. This can be anywhere from three weeks to three months depending on the program. It is common for therapists to use SI treatment techniques within their sessions alongside other treatment tools.

The intensity is a key component of creating the neurological changes necessary to facilitate neuroplasticity.

Good treatment is the result of a comprehensive assessment. We must know what we are looking at to build the most appropriate plan. A builder doesn't start a house with the walls, he throws a foundation first according to the plans of the finished house. So too, as therapists, we must have a strong foundation from which to develop the treatment plan.

The plan follows the principals of brain development and hierarchical structures.

The goal of treatment is to ensure that we are filling the gaps that were created when the sensory systems developed maladaptive responses to maintain a perceived sense of safety; by encouraging new patterns of development using this step-up approach.

Treatment focuses on the first level of Sensory Processing: body-spatial awareness, discrimination, self-regulation and protection.

Level 2: Visual perception incorporates integrating visual, auditory and vestibular processing. This ensures that the highly complex visual system is addressed before moving onto higher level motor skills.

Level 3: Co-ordination incorporates visual motor integration, postural control and bilateral integration. Co-ordination requires good communication between the right and left sides of the brain. This communication relies on connections that are built in the deep structures of the brain. When these connections are limited, gross motor co-ordination, tone, hip and shoulder stability are generally poor resulting in slow developing motor skills.

Speech relies on motor co-ordination of the tongue and facial muscles so when there is weakness in the muscles and connection activity, there is definite weakness in tongue, lip and facial muscle development resulting in expressive language delays, articulation difficulties and picky eating.

Level 4: The Communication level includes oral motor development, expressive and receptive language and auditory processing.

Intensive Step up Approach to Intervention

Therapeutic Step Program
(The Children's Therapy Works Approach)

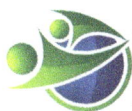

Sensory Processing	Visual Perception	Coordination	Communication	Function	Goal
Body/Spatial Awareness	Visual	Visual Motor Integration	Oral Motor (Articulation/Feeding)	Refined Skills	**Academics**
Discrimination	Auditory		Expressive Language		
Self-Regulation	Vestibular	Postural Control	Receptive Language	Pragmatics	
Protection		Bilateral Integration	Auditory Processing	Activities of Daily Living	

ACADEMY
AT NORTH FULTON

4/14/2014

© 1998-2014 Children's Therapy Works

Speech and language is a cognitive skill that relies on so many facets of brain development that it is one of the last skills to develop. This is why it is one of the last levels that we work on. By the time we reach this level, the child has usually mastered many skills themselves because all the pieces are falling into place. By the time we reach this point in an intensive, we are starting to work on refining skills and creating new ones depending on how old the child is.

These building blocks all lead to improving functional activities of daily living. Function involves refining motor skills such as writing development or playing with puzzles or blocks.

Pragmatic language involves concept formation and social skills and activities of daily living skills require complex integration and organization of a number of skills that are needed to form routines to manage time that allows for building complex skills and proficiency.

This is where developmental charts are helpful, but remember, every child develops individually and we cannot always depend on such definite, concrete stages to define where the child is in their development.

We use these developmental milestones as guidelines for goal development and helping determine what the baseline points are to begin with. This bottom up approach promotes development without necessarily working on that specific skill over and over again. Repetition doesn't create a new skill — it can develop into a splinter skill, which means that there is a specific skill that a child can perform but it can't be translated into regular life.

Our objective is to fill the holes so that the child can discover their own creative, well organized, efficient way of learning that constructs new patterns of development. Once these patterns become established, learning breakthroughs occur consistently for months after the intensive therapies are reduced.

Once neuroplasticity occurs, we can see the changes globally. This child is capable of translating various skills into different situations and environments more successfully. This is when practice becomes important to hone in on a skill and improve the quality and quantity of how it is done.

Chapter 8

So what do I do now?

So now what? There is nothing more stressful as a parent than not knowing how to help your child. There are so many parenting books out today on behavior, cognitive development, and autism, ADD etc. How do you know what to look for? What does a good therapist look like? How do I know if my child is getting the right therapy. Well, being a parent did not come with the manual, however I am a big believer in gut feel. Trust your instinct and allow your child to tell you what they need. Listen! Listen to the cues your child is giving you and hear what they are saying — that's what a good occupational, speech and physical therapist does as well. They listen and integrate information for you to think about and try. They make your job a little easier as parent by giving you strategies that can be used in all settings so the learning can be carried through into all environments.

Let's start here

If you suspect that your child may be struggling with something, or your toddler is not speaking yet and seems to be falling behind, ask your pediatrician for a referral to an Occupational therapist and Speech therapist for an assessment. Many pediatricians will tell you to wait and not to worry, that your child is just a late bloomer — if you are concerned, insist on the script. I tell parents all the time that I would rather rule out any issues early on, then wait for them to become a huge problem. It is YOUR decision to go for an evaluation. Just FYI, you do not need a Doctor's script for the evaluation for occupational therapy — you do need one for treatment however and to get insurance to cover the therapy if it is needed.

The process should go like this

1. Talk to pediatrician and get a script
2. Look for an occupational therapist that specializes in sensory integration.
3. Schedule an evaluation to determine whether there are specific areas of difficulty.
4. Participate in an intensive program to make changes quickly and effectively.

Sounds simple right? It can be.

In the therapy world, occupational therapists are usually the therapists trained in sensory integration treatment — however there are some incredible speech and physical therapists that have also gone through SIPT certification.

A little more info about assessments

The Sensory Integration and Praxis Test (SIPT) is the gold standard for evaluating whether a child has sensory integration dysfunction. The test is standardized for children between the ages of four years —

eight years 11 months. After that, the test may be used in special circumstances but the standardization sample will not be within range.

The SIPT correlates highly to IQ testing, speech testing scores and psychological tests. This is why it is such an excellent tool from which to gain information.

For younger children, we have some great options that look at functional sensory processing skills through parent checklists and measuring motor and language skill development. These are typically screening tools and with good clinical observations, a trained therapist can address the needs of a younger child.

Some examples of these include

The Sensory Profile, Sensory Processing Measure, School Function Assessment, Sensory checklists, Clinical Observations and more.

Another tool that we use in our practice is called the Brain Map—this is a mini EEG that tells us how the brain waves are accessing cortical information. It is also highly effective for determining which programs to focus on in order to achieve the "bottom-up" approach to filling in gaps.

The Brain Map is exactly that — it maps out and correlates how much energy the alpha, beta, theta, delta waves have to use in higher cortical areas of the brain.

The Brain map is a powerful tool that answers many questions for both therapists and parents as it makes everything very visual and tangible. It also aligns closely to the testing results from the SIPT and psychological evaluations.

By understanding how all these results interrelate, we are able to pinpoint which area to start with — is the body spatial awareness creating the block or does the child struggle with self regulation?

By understanding the brain maps, we can identify where to start treatment.

The four primary brain waves control our "mental state," but what controls the brainwaves?

The myriad of chemicals and electrical impulses create energetic transfer. There is so much information about energy today — the TV stations are now making mini-series of the different ways that energy is understood today.

The facts are that electrical activity in the brain has to be efficiently moved between neurons in order for an impulse to fire and a nerve and synapse to respond. Well if this energy is not accessible because it is being used else where in the brain to keep the brain safe, then we see this on the brain map as a high or low response.

Conclusion

A conclusion is always difficult to write! As there is so much to tell you about sensory processing and children. What I can add to this discussion is that in 2010, we began building a pilot program for a school using all these techniques and theories. At the time that I am writing, we are four years down the line and the school is proving these theories! We have children with varying diagnoses and ages that couldn't function in other learning environments or were asked to leave for various reasons. We are at the end of our school year and have just finished testing — the results speak for themselves! All our students have made academic improvements of up to 65%, with the lowest score being 35%. Not only am I proud of my teams but watching these children grow from being scared, angry, confused little beings into self directed, verbal, empowered children — well words can't really express that emotion! And for those of you who know me, know that I cry every time I talk about these kids achievements — because that's what makes it all worthwhile!

I will leave you with a little story.

In April of 2014, a couple of months before finishing this book, I received a call from one of my long time colleagues. She asked me if I remembered this child that we treated about 15 years ago. I'm usually pretty good about remembering my clients, but for some reason, this was a little guy that I couldn't place. Sharon asked me if I would be willing to write a letter explaining to the school he was attending, what Motor Dyspraxia was. "Sure!"

I replied and agreed to see the client who was coming from out of town on the following Monday.

I was very excited to see this client, it's always inspiring seeing our kids grow up, but nothing prepared me for what came next.

This tall, good looking, 6'2," full bearded MAN walked into my office with his mom on the Monday morning — I recognized the mom, but definitely didn't recognize him. So a little background on JP — as a young child, he was diagnosed with speech apraxia (difficulty learning and expressing himself). He was non verbal when he came to us and had pretty severe Co-ordination difficulties too. While we were chit chatting and catching up, he told me that when he was verbalizing, he thought he was talking and he could not understand why nobody responded to him. What we were hearing, was a child making screeching noises without any order or form to the sounds. To everyone else, JP was a screamer, to JP, he was trying to communicate. After some intense therapies, he went to school and we didn't see him again until now — at age 19.

JP had reached a point in his life where

he knew he needed a little help with learning. You see part of the dyspraxia diagnosis is that the brain translates information differently so, he was having trouble taking notes and listening to the lecturer at the same time. He just needed a few accommodations for note taking and test taking in order to keep up with the rigors of college — oh, did I forget to mention? JP had been accepted into Johns Hopkins medical school. He was studying to be a doctor..... who specialized in neurology!

Hey Mrs. Shelley,

Thank you for seeing me last week, it was great seeing you. I have included my testimony below. Every word is the truth and I hope it can help. Also when you get a chance, can you please send the letter you wrote for me to this email? I am trying to meet with the director Monday if possible. Thanks for all that you have done and I look forward to working with you in the summer.

When I was diagnosed with Apraxia as a child, I discovered that my condition affected me in other areas besides my ability to speak. Most notably I was very susceptible to being overwhelmed by sensory stimulation and had difficulty performing gross and fine motor skills essential to a normal life. To compensate for this, my parents took me to Children's Therapy Works. With their expertise and assistance I have been able to not only achieve the skills needed for adulthood but also go far beyond to achieve things I never thought possible. I am currently playing football at Johns Hopkins University, which without CTW would have been impossible. J-P

CHILDREN'S THERAPY WORKS
Glossary

Sensory Integration Terminology

Page Brunner, OTS
Brenau University

Adaptive Response: An appropriate response to an environmental demand. Adaptive responses demonstrate adequate sensory integration and drive all learning and social interactions.

Auditory Perception: The ability to receive, identify, discriminate, understand and respond to sounds.

Bilateral Coordination: The ability to use both sides of the body together in a smooth, synchronized, and coordinated manner.

Is this my child?

Bilateral Integration: The neurological process of integrating sensations from both body sides; the foundation for bilateral coordination.

Body Awareness: The identifying of one's own body parts: where they are, how they interrelate, and how they move.

Co-contraction: All muscle groups surrounding a joint contracting and working together to provide joint stability, resulting in the ability to maintain position and balance.

Depth Perception: The ability to judge relative distances between objects, or between oneself and objects. Also affects ability to see objects in three dimensions.

Directionality: The awareness of directions (right/left, forward/back, and up/down), and the ability to move oneself in those directions.

Discriminative System: The component of a sensory system that allows one to identify differences among stimuli. This system is not innate but develops with time and practice.

Dyspraxia: Difficulty in planning, sequencing, and carrying out unfamiliar actions in a skillful manner. Poor motor planning is the result of dyspraxia.
Eye-Hand Coordination: The efficient teamwork of

the eyes and hands, necessary for activities such as playing with toys, dressing, and writing.

Equilibrium: A term used to mean balance.

Extension: A straightening action of a joint (neck, back, arms, legs).

Fight-Or-Flight Response: The instinctive reaction to defend oneself from real or perceived danger by becoming aggressive or by withdrawing.

Figure-Ground Perception: The ability to perceive a figure in the foreground from a rival background.

Fine Motor: Referring to refined movement of the muscles in the fingers, toes, eyes and tongue.

Fine Motor Skills: The skilled use of one's hands in a smooth, precise and controlled manner. Fine motor control is essential for efficient handling of classroom tools and materials. It may also be referred to as dexterity.

Fixation: The ability to aim one's eye at an object and maintain gaze or shifting one's gaze from one object to another.

Flexion: A bending action of a joint or a pulling in of a body part.

Is this my child?

Form Constancy: Recognition of a shape regardless of its size, position, or texture.

Gravitational Insecurity: The fear and anxiety of falling when one's head position changes.

Gross Motor: Movements of the large muscles of the body.

Gross Motor Skills: Coordinated body movements involving the large muscle groups. Activities requiring this skill include running, walking, hopping, climbing, throwing and jumping.

Habituation: The neurological process which allows the tuning out of familiar sensations.

Hand Preference: Right - or left handedness, which becomes established in childhood as early as the age of 3, however does not become well established until the age of 8 or 9.

Hypersensitivity: (also Hyper-reactivity or Hyper-responsiveness). Oversensitivity to sensory stimuli, characterized by a tendency to be either fearful and cautious, or negative and defiant.

Hyposensitivity: (also Hyporeactivity or Hyporesponsiveness). Undersensitivity to sensory stimuli, characterized by a tendency either to crave intense sensations or to withdraw and be difficult to engage.

Kinesthesia: The conscious awareness of joint position and body movement in space, such as knowing where to place one's feet when climbing stairs, without visual cues.

Lateralization: The process of establishing preference of one side of the brain for directing skilled motor function on the opposite side of the body, while the opposite side is used for stabilization. Lateralization is necessary for establishing hand preference and crossing the body midline.

Linear movement: A motion in which one moves in a line, from front to back, side to side, or up and down.

Low Tone: The lack of supportive muscle tone, usually with increased mobility at the joints; the person with low tone seems "loose and floppy."

Midline: A median line dividing the two halves of the body. Crossing the midline is the ability to use one side or part of the body (hand, foot, or eye) in the space of the other side or part.

Modulation: The brain's ability to regulate its own activity.

Motor Control: The ability to regulate the motions of one's muscle groups in order to work together harmoniously to perform movements.

Is this my child?

Motor Coordination: The ability of several muscles or muscle groups to work together harmoniously to perform movements.

Motor Planning: The ability to conceive of, organize, sequence, and carry out an unfamiliar or complex body movement in a coordinated manner, a component of praxis.

Muscle Tone: The degree of tension normally present when one's muscles are relaxed, or in a resting state.

Perception: The meaning the brain attributes to sensory input.

Plasticity: The ability of the brain to change or to be changed as a result of activity, especially as one responds to sensations.

Position in Space: Awareness of the spatial orientation of letters, words, numbers, or drawings on a page, or of an object in the environment.

Postural Adjustments: The ability to shift one's body in order to change position for a task.

Postural Insecurity: A fear of body movement that is related to poor balance, and deficient "body and spatial" awareness.

Postural Stability: The ability to maintain one's body in a position to efficiently complete a task or demand, using large muscle groups at the shoulders and hips.

Praxis: Praxis is a broad term denoting voluntary and coordinated action. The ability to interact successfully with the physical environment; to plan, organize, and carry out a sequence of unfamiliar actions; and to do what one needs and wants to do. Motor planning is often a used as a synonym.
Prone: A horizontal position of the body where the face is positioned downward.

Proprioception: The unconscious awareness of sensations coming from one's joints, muscles, tendons, and ligaments that aids in knowing where one is in space; the "position sense."

Rotary Movement: turning or spinning in circles.
Self-Care Skills: Competence in taking care of one's personal needs, such as bathing, dressing, eating, and grooming.

Self-Regulation: The ability to control one's activity level and state of alertness, as well as one's emotional, mental or physical responses to senses; self-organization.

Sensorimotor: Pertaining to the brain-behavior of taking in sensory messages and reacting with a physical response.

Is this my child?

Sensory Defensiveness: A child's behavior in response to sensory input, reflecting severe over-reactions or a low threshold to a specific sensory input.

Sensory Diet: The multisensory experiences that one normally seeks on a daily basis to satisfy one's sensory appetite; a planned and scheduled activity program that an occupational therapist develops to help a person become more self-regulated.

Sensory Input: The constant flow of information from sensory receptors in the body to the brain and spinal cord.

Sensory Integration: The normal neurological process taking in information from one's body and environment through the senses, of organizing and unifying this information, and using it to plan and execute adaptive responses to different challenges in order to learn and function smoothly in daily life.

Sensory Integrative Dysfunction: The inefficient neurological processing of information received through the senses, causing problems with learning, development and behavior.

Sensory Integration Theory: A concept based on neurology, research and behavior that explains the brain-behavior relationship.

Sensory Integration Treatment: A technique of occupational therapy, which provides playful, meaningful activities that enhance an individual's sensory intake and lead to more adaptive functioning in daily life.

Sensory Modulation: Maintenance of the arousal state to generate emotional responses, sustain attention, develop appropriate activity level and move skillfully.

Sensory Processing Skills: The ability to receive and process information from one's sensory systems including touch (tactile), visual, auditory (hearing), proprioceptive (body position) and vestibular (balance). Behavior, attention and peer interactions are greatly influenced by the child's ability to process sensory stimuli.

Sensory Registration: Initial awareness of a single input.

Sensory Threshold: The level of strength a stimulus must reach in order to be detected. This is the mechanism that drives our reactions to sensory input and whether we over-react or under-register the input.

Spatial Awareness: The perception of one's proximity to or distance from an object, as well as the perception of the relationship of one's body parts.

Supine: A horizontal body position where the face is positioned upward.

Tactile: Refers to the sense of touch and various qualities attributed to touch: including detecting pressure, temperature, light touch, pain, discriminative touch.

Tactile Defensiveness: The tendency to react negatively and emotionally to unexpected. Light touch sensations.

Tracking: Following a moving object or a line of print with the eyes.

Vestibular: The sensory system that responds to changes in head and body movement through space, and that coordinates movements of the eyes, head, and body. Receptor site is in the inner ear. Gravitational Insecurity is a function of the vestibular system.

Visual Discrimination: Differentiating among symbols and forms, such as matching or separating colors, shapes, numbers, letters, and words.

Visual Figure-Ground: Differentiation between objects in the foreground and in the background
Visual-Motor: Referring to one's movements based on the perception of visual information.

Visual Motor Skills: The ability to visually take in information, process it and be able to coordinate your physical movement in relation to what has been viewed. It involves the combination of visual perception and motor coordination. Difficulty with visual motor skills can result in inaccurate reaching, pointing and grasping of objects, as well as difficulty with copying, drawing, tracing and cutting.

Visual-Perception: The ability to perceive and interpret what the eyes see.

Visual Perceptual Skills: The ability to interpret and use what is seen in the environment. Difficulties in this area can interfere with a child's ability to learn self-help skills like tying shoelaces and academic tasks like copying from the blackboard or finding items in a busy background.

Visual-Spatial Processing Skills: Perceptions based on sensory information received through the eyes and body as one interacts with the environment and moves one's body through space. Including: Depth perception, directionality, form constancy, position in space, spatial awareness, visual discrimination, visual figure-ground.

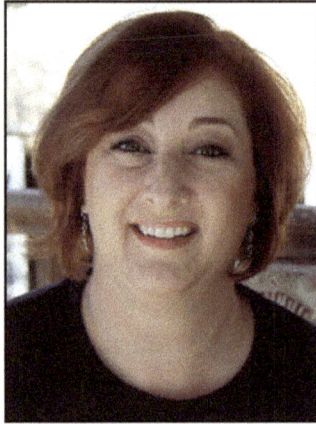

Shelley Margow MS.OTR/L is the owner and clinical director of Children's Therapy Works, a pediatric private practice in Roswell, Georgia. She earned a Bachelor of Science degree in Occupational Therapy at the University of the Witwatersrand in Johannesburg, South Africa and received her Post-Professional Masters Degree from Sargent College at Boston University. Mrs. Margow has certifications in: Sensory Integration and Praxis Test, Samonas Sound Therapy, Sensory Learning Program, Fast ForWord, and Integrated Listening Systems.

In 1998, she opened Children's Therapy Works, an industry leader in providing therapeutic programming for children who have difficulty functioning at home, at school, or within their community. Their services include Occupational, Speech, and Physical Therapy, utilizing a multidisciplinary approach, sensory integration and neurodevelopmental tools specific to each individual and family. The philosophy of the clinic focuses on using intensive, neurological treatment to facilitate brain plasticity.

In 2010, she started a pilot school to meet the needs of children with Dyspraxia, Learning Disabilities, Autism spectrum disorders and more. Now named the Academy at North Fulton, the accredited, non-profit school provides innovative, integrated, and top-quality therapeutic services for grades K-12, addressing and facilitating the child's most effective way of learning, and helping establish the confidence they need to progress in an academic setting.

Ms. Margow has developed training programs for occupational, speech and physical therapists and published articles for Georgia Occupational Therapy Association, local magazines and online media. She has lectured therapists, teachers and parents on integrating sensory integration and oral-motor techniques. Ms. Margow has also presented at the National Down Syndrome Congress and at the Autism Avenue: 2013 Regional "Possibilities & Potential" Autism/Asperger Conference. She was recently featured as a "She'ro" in the North Fulton Women's Magazine (December 2013) and again in the January edition.

www.ingramcontent.com/pod-product-compliance
Lightning Source LLC
Chambersburg PA
CBHW051247020426
42333CB00025B/3101